Table Of Contents

Chapter 1: Understanding Binge Eating

What is Binge Eating?

Binge eating is a serious condition that affects many individuals who struggle with out of control eating habits. It is characterized by consuming large amounts of food in a short period of time, often to the point of discomfort or pain. People who binge eat may feel a loss of control over their eating and may eat alone in secret, feeling ashamed or guilty about their behavior.

Binge eating is not simply overeating or indulging in a large meal on occasion. It is a pattern of behavior that can have serious physical and emotional consequences. Those who struggle with binge eating may use food as a way to cope with stress, anxiety, or other negative emotions, leading to a cycle of guilt, shame, and further binge eating.

If you find yourself unable to stop eating, feeling like you have no control over your food intake, and eating in secret, it is important to seek help. Binge eating disorder is a recognized mental health condition that can be treated with therapy, support groups, and sometimes medication. It is important to remember that you are not alone in your struggle and that there is help available.

Breaking the Binge: A Guide to Overcoming Out of Control Eating offers practical tips and strategies for addressing binge eating behavior. By learning to recognize triggers, practicing mindfulness, and developing healthy coping mechanisms, you can begin to regain control over your eating habits and improve your overall well-being. Remember, it is never too late to seek help and make positive changes in your life.

The Cycle of Binge Eating

Binge eating can often feel like an endless cycle that is impossible to break. For many individuals who struggle with out of control eating, the urge to consume large amounts of food can be overwhelming and all-consuming. This cycle of binge eating can lead to feelings of guilt, shame, and hopelessness, creating a vicious cycle that is difficult to escape.

The first step in breaking the cycle of binge eating is to understand the triggers that lead to episodes of overeating. These triggers can vary from person to person and may include stress, boredom, loneliness, or even feelings of deprivation. By identifying these triggers, individuals can begin to develop coping strategies to address them in a healthier way.

One common trigger for binge eating is emotional distress. Many individuals turn to food as a way to cope with difficult emotions or to numb themselves from feelings of sadness, loneliness, or anxiety. By finding alternative ways to manage these emotions, such as through therapy, mindfulness practices, or engaging in enjoyable activities, individuals can begin to break the cycle of using food as a crutch.

Another important aspect of breaking the cycle of binge eating is to create a supportive environment. This may involve reaching out to loved ones for help, seeking support from a therapist or support group, or finding healthy outlets for stress relief. By surrounding oneself with a positive support system, individuals can begin to feel less isolated and more empowered to make positive changes in their eating habits.

Ultimately, breaking the cycle of binge eating requires self-awareness, commitment, and perseverance. By taking small steps towards understanding the root causes of overeating and developing healthier coping mechanisms, individuals can begin to regain control over their eating habits and break free from the cycle of binge eating. Remember, you are not alone in this journey, and there is always help and support available to guide you towards a healthier relationship with food.

Signs and Symptoms of Binge Eating Disorder

Binge Eating Disorder (BED) is a serious condition that affects many individuals who struggle with out of control eating habits. Recognizing the signs and symptoms of BED is the first step towards seeking help and overcoming this challenging disorder.

One of the most common signs of BED is consuming large amounts of food in a short period of time, often to the point of feeling uncomfortably full. People with BED may also experience feelings of guilt, shame, or distress after a binge episode. They may try to hide their eating habits from others, eating in secret or when alone to avoid judgment or scrutiny.

Another key symptom of BED is a lack of control over eating behaviors. Individuals with this disorder may feel like they cannot stop eating, even when they are physically full or when they know they should stop. This feeling of being unable to control their eating can lead to cycles of bingeing and restriction, which can have serious consequences for both physical and mental health.

It is important for individuals struggling with BED to seek support and treatment from a qualified healthcare professional. Therapy, support groups, and nutritional counseling can all be helpful in addressing the underlying issues that contribute to binge eating behaviors. By learning to identify triggers, develop healthier coping mechanisms, and build a more positive relationship with food, individuals with BED can work towards breaking the cycle of binge eating and reclaiming control over their eating habits.

Chapter 2: The Impact of Out of Control Eating

Physical Health Consequences

The physical health consequences of binge eating and out of control eating can be detrimental to your overall well-being. When you constantly consume large amounts of food in a short period of time, it can lead to weight gain, obesity, and a host of other health issues.

One of the main concerns with binge eating is the potential for developing cardiovascular problems such as high blood pressure, high cholesterol, and an increased risk of heart disease. The excess calories and unhealthy foods consumed during binges can also contribute to the development of type 2 diabetes.

In addition to the increased risk of chronic diseases, binge eating can also have negative effects on your digestive system. Eating large quantities of food can overload your stomach and intestines, leading to discomfort, bloating, and indigestion. This can also disrupt your body's natural hunger and fullness cues, making it even harder to control your eating habits.

Furthermore, binge eating can have a significant impact on your mental health. Feelings of guilt, shame, and low self-esteem can arise from the lack of control over your eating habits, leading to a vicious cycle of emotional eating and further binge episodes.

If you find yourself unable to stop eating mindlessly and alone, it is important to seek help and support. Consider reaching out to a therapist or counselor who specializes in eating disorders, or joining a support group for individuals struggling with binge eating. By addressing the underlying emotional issues and developing healthier coping mechanisms, you can begin to regain control over your eating habits and improve your physical and mental well-being.

Emotional and Mental Health Effects

The emotional and mental health effects of binge eating can be profound and far-reaching. For those who cannot stop eating and have no control over their food intake, the shame, guilt, and self-loathing that often accompany binge eating can be overwhelming. The secrecy and isolation that often come with binge eating can also have a detrimental impact on mental health, leading to feelings of loneliness and despair.

Many people who struggle with binge eating find themselves caught in a vicious cycle of using food as a coping mechanism for dealing with negative emotions such as stress, anxiety, or depression. However, this only serves to exacerbate the problem, as the temporary relief provided by food is quickly replaced by feelings of guilt and shame.

In addition to the emotional toll, binge eating can also have serious implications for mental health. Research has shown that binge eating is often linked to other mental health disorders such as depression, anxiety, and low self-esteem. Left unchecked, binge eating can lead to a host of physical health problems, including obesity, heart disease, and diabetes.

If you find yourself unable to stop eating mindlessly and are struggling with out-of-control eating, it is important to seek help. There are a variety of resources available, including therapy, support groups, and self-help books like this one, that can provide you with the tools and strategies you need to overcome binge eating and regain control over your eating habits. Remember, you are not alone, and there is help available to support you on your journey to breaking the binge.

Social and Relationship Impacts

The social and relationship impacts of binge eating can be profound and far-reaching. For those who struggle with out-of-control eating in secret, the isolation and shame can be overwhelming. Many people find themselves hiding their binge eating behaviors from family and friends, leading to feelings of guilt and embarrassment. This can create a cycle of shame and secrecy that only serves to perpetuate the problem.

In addition to the emotional toll, binge eating can also have negative effects on relationships. Loved ones may become concerned or frustrated by the behavior, leading to strained relationships and misunderstandings. People who struggle with binge eating may also isolate themselves from social situations out of fear of judgment or embarrassment. This can further exacerbate feelings of loneliness and isolation.

Breaking free from the cycle of binge eating requires reaching out for help and support. It's important for individuals struggling with out-of-control eating to know that they are not alone and that there are resources available to help them overcome their challenges. Seeking help from a therapist or counselor who specializes in eating disorders can be a crucial first step in breaking the cycle of binge eating.

Building a support network of understanding friends and family members can also be beneficial. Opening up about struggles with binge eating can be difficult, but it can also be a powerful step toward healing and recovery. By sharing their experiences and seeking support, individuals struggling with binge eating can begin to break free from the cycle of shame and isolation and start on the path to a healthier relationship with food and themselves.

Chapter 3: Factors Contributing to Binge Eating

Genetics and Biology

Genetics and biology play a significant role in our eating behaviors, particularly for those who struggle with binge eating and have no control over their food intake. Research has shown that certain genetic factors can predispose individuals to develop unhealthy eating patterns, such as a tendency to overeat or a heightened sensitivity to food cues.

Additionally, our biology can also influence our eating habits. Hormones like ghrelin, which signals hunger, and leptin, which signals fullness, can impact our appetite and satiety levels. Imbalances in these hormones can lead to increased cravings and a difficulty in feeling satisfied after eating, contributing to the cycle of binge eating.

Understanding the genetic and biological factors at play can help individuals struggling with out of control eating to have more compassion for themselves. It is not simply a lack of willpower or self-control that drives their behaviors, but rather a complex interplay of genetics and biology that can make it difficult to resist the urge to overeat.

While genetics and biology may contribute to the development of binge eating behaviors, it is important to remember that these are not determinants of one's destiny. With the right support and tools, individuals can learn to overcome their urges to binge eat and develop healthier eating habits.

In the next sections of this book, we will explore practical strategies and techniques to help individuals break free from the cycle of binge eating and regain control over their food intake. By understanding the role of genetics and biology in their eating behaviors, individuals can take the first step towards making positive changes in their relationship with food.

Psychological Factors

One of the key components to understanding and overcoming out of control eating is recognizing the psychological factors that contribute to this behavior. Many individuals who struggle with binge eating or out of control eating often do so in secret, feeling shame and guilt about their inability to stop. It is important to address these psychological factors in order to break the cycle of mindless eating.

One common psychological factor that contributes to out of control eating is emotional eating. Many people turn to food as a way to cope with difficult emotions such as stress, anxiety, or loneliness. This can lead to a pattern of using food as a form of self-soothing, which only perpetuates the problem.

Another psychological factor that can contribute to out of control eating is a lack of mindfulness. Mindful eating involves being present and aware of the food you are consuming, as well as your body's hunger and fullness cues. When individuals eat mindlessly, they are more likely to overeat without even realizing it.

It is important for individuals struggling with out of control eating to address these psychological factors in order to make lasting changes. Seeking support from a therapist or counselor can be helpful in uncovering the underlying issues that contribute to this behavior. Additionally, practicing mindfulness techniques such as deep breathing, meditation, or yoga can help individuals become more aware of their eating habits and make healthier choices.

By addressing the psychological factors that contribute to out of control eating, individuals can begin to break free from the cycle of mindless eating and regain control over their relationship with food. It is important to remember that seeking help and support is not a sign of weakness, but rather a brave step towards overcoming this challenging behavior.

Environmental Triggers

Environmental triggers play a significant role in perpetuating the cycle of binge eating and out-of-control eating. These triggers can be both internal and external, and understanding them is crucial in overcoming mindless eating habits.

Internal triggers may include emotions such as stress, anxiety, boredom, or loneliness. When we are feeling overwhelmed or distressed, we may turn to food as a way to cope with these feelings. It provides a temporary sense of comfort and distraction from our emotions, leading to a cycle of emotional eating.

External triggers, on the other hand, are environmental factors that can stimulate the urge to eat excessively. These triggers may include the presence of food cues like TV commercials, food advertisements, or the smell of food in the environment. Social situations, such as parties or gatherings, can also trigger overeating as we may feel pressure to indulge or overeat in the presence of others.

To break free from the grip of environmental triggers, it is essential to first identify them. Keeping a food diary can help you track your eating patterns and identify the triggers that lead to mindless eating episodes. Once you have identified your triggers, you can develop strategies to avoid or cope with them.

Creating a supportive environment is also key in overcoming out-of-control eating. Surround yourself with people who understand and respect your journey towards healthier eating habits. Communicate your needs and boundaries with those around you to ensure that you are not tempted by triggers in your environment.

By recognizing and addressing environmental triggers, you can take the first step towards breaking the cycle of binge eating and reclaiming control over your eating habits. Remember, you are not alone in this journey, and with the right support and strategies, you can overcome mindless eating and create a healthier relationship with food.

Chapter 4: Overcoming Binge Eating

Seeking Professional Help

Seeking professional help is a crucial step in overcoming out of control eating habits. If you find yourself constantly eating in secret, feeling like you have no control over your eating, and struggling to stop mindlessly consuming food, it may be time to seek the guidance of a trained professional.

Therapists, counselors, and nutritionists specializing in eating disorders can provide you with the support and tools you need to break free from the cycle of binge eating. These professionals can help you identify the underlying emotional issues that may be driving your eating behaviors and develop coping strategies to manage them effectively.

Cognitive-behavioral therapy (CBT) is a commonly used approach for treating binge eating disorder. This type of therapy helps individuals recognize and challenge their negative thought patterns and develop healthier ways of coping with stress and emotions. CBT can also help you learn to identify triggers for binge eating and develop strategies to manage them.

In addition to therapy, working with a nutritionist can help you establish a balanced and healthy relationship with food. A nutritionist can help you create a meal plan that meets your nutritional needs while also addressing your emotional relationship with food. They can also provide guidance on mindful eating techniques and help you develop a healthier approach to food and eating.

Remember, seeking professional help is not a sign of weakness, but a courageous step towards reclaiming control over your eating habits and your life. Don't be afraid to reach out for support – you deserve to live a life free from the burden of out of control eating.

Developing Healthy Coping Mechanisms

Developing Healthy Coping Mechanisms is crucial for individuals struggling with binge eating and out of control eating. It is common for those dealing with these issues to turn to food as a form of comfort or escape from negative emotions. However, there are healthier ways to cope with stress, anxiety, and other triggers that may lead to overeating.

One effective coping mechanism is mindfulness. Mindful eating involves paying attention to the sensations of eating, such as the taste, texture, and smell of food. By being present in the moment while eating, individuals can better tune into their body's hunger and fullness cues, helping to prevent mindless overeating.

Another helpful coping mechanism is finding alternative ways to manage emotions. This could include engaging in activities such as exercise, journaling, meditation, or talking to a therapist. By finding healthy outlets for emotions, individuals can reduce the urge to turn to food for comfort.

It is also important to create a supportive environment. This may involve reaching out to friends, family members, or a support group for encouragement and accountability. Having someone to talk to about struggles with food can make a big difference in breaking the cycle of binge eating.

Overall, developing healthy coping mechanisms is essential for overcoming out of control eating. By practicing mindfulness, finding alternative ways to manage emotions, and creating a supportive environment, individuals can begin to break free from the cycle of binge eating and regain control over their eating habits.

Building a Support System

Building a support system is crucial for individuals struggling with out-of-control eating habits. Whether you are binge eating in secret or constantly overeating when no one is around, having a strong support system can make all the difference in overcoming this challenging behavior.

The first step in building a support system is acknowledging that you need help. It can be difficult to open up about your struggles with food, especially if you have been keeping them hidden for a long time. However, reaching out for support is the first step towards healing and recovery.

One way to build a support system is to confide in a trusted friend or family member. Opening up about your struggles with out-of-control eating can be scary, but having someone to confide in can provide much-needed emotional support and understanding. This person can also help hold you accountable and provide encouragement as you work towards breaking free from your unhealthy eating habits.

Another important aspect of building a support system is seeking professional help. Consider reaching out to a therapist or counselor who specializes in eating disorders. They can help you understand the root causes of your out-of-control eating and provide you with tools and strategies to overcome it.

Joining a support group for individuals struggling with binge eating or out-of-control eating can also be incredibly beneficial. Connecting with others who are going through similar experiences can provide a sense of community and understanding that is key to recovery.

Remember, you don't have to face your struggles with food alone. Building a support system of understanding friends, family, professionals, and peers can help you on your journey towards breaking free from out-of-control eating habits and living a healthier, more balanced life.

Chapter 5: Mindful Eating Practices

Being Present in the Moment

Being present in the moment is a crucial tool in overcoming out of control eating and binge eating. Many people who struggle with these issues find themselves mindlessly consuming food, often in isolation and without anyone else knowing. It can feel like an uncontrollable urge that takes over, leaving individuals feeling powerless and ashamed.

One way to combat this behavior is to practice mindfulness and be fully present in the moment when eating. This means paying attention to your thoughts, feelings, and sensations without judgment. By being aware of your emotions and triggers, you can start to understand why you turn to food as a coping mechanism.

Mindful eating involves slowing down and savoring each bite, acknowledging the taste, texture, and smell of the food. It also involves listening to your body's hunger and fullness cues, eating when you are truly hungry and stopping when you are satisfied. By being present in the moment, you can better recognize when you are eating out of habit or emotional need rather than true hunger.

Incorporating mindfulness practices such as deep breathing, meditation, or yoga can also help you become more attuned to your body and emotions, making it easier to resist the urge to binge eat. By being present and mindful in your eating habits, you can break the cycle of out of control eating and develop a healthier relationship with food. Remember, you are not alone in this struggle, and there are resources and support available to help you on your journey to recovery.

Listening to Your Body's Hunger Cues

One of the key steps in overcoming out of control eating is learning to listen to your body's hunger cues. Many individuals who struggle with binge eating often ignore or suppress their body's signals of hunger and fullness, leading to mindless and excessive eating. By tuning in to what your body is telling you, you can begin to regain control over your eating habits and break free from the cycle of binge eating.

Start by paying attention to physical signs of hunger, such as stomach growling, lightheadedness, or feeling fatigued. These are signals that your body needs nourishment and it is important to respond to them in a healthy way. Instead of reaching for the nearest high-calorie snack, take a moment to assess your hunger level and choose nutritious foods that will satisfy you.

Similarly, it is crucial to recognize when you are full and stop eating when you are satisfied. This can be challenging for individuals who struggle with binge eating, as they may feel compelled to continue eating even when they are no longer hungry. Practice mindful eating by slowing down, savoring each bite, and checking in with your body throughout the meal. By listening to your body's cues, you can prevent overeating and feel more in tune with your natural hunger and fullness signals.

Incorporating regular meal times, planning balanced meals, and keeping a food journal can also help you stay attuned to your body's needs and prevent mindless eating. Remember, breaking the binge cycle starts with listening to your body and honoring its signals of hunger and fullness. With practice and patience, you can regain control over your eating habits and find freedom from out of control eating.

Practicing Self-Compassion

Practicing self-compassion is a crucial step in overcoming out of control eating habits. Many people who struggle with binge eating do so in isolation, feeling ashamed and alone in their struggles. However, it is important to remember that you are not alone in this battle and that self-compassion can be a powerful tool in breaking the cycle of binge eating.

Self-compassion involves treating yourself with kindness and understanding, rather than harsh criticism and judgment. This means acknowledging that you are human and that everyone makes mistakes, including overeating. Instead of beating yourself up for giving in to your cravings, try to approach yourself with compassion and understanding.

One way to practice self-compassion is to speak to yourself as you would to a close friend who is struggling. Would you berate your friend for overeating, or would you offer them support and encouragement? Treat yourself with the same kindness and understanding that you would show to a friend in need.

Another important aspect of self-compassion is to practice mindfulness. This involves being present in the moment and paying attention to your thoughts and feelings without judgment. When you feel the urge to binge eat, take a moment to pause and check in with yourself. Ask yourself what you are truly hungry for, whether it is food or something else, such as comfort or emotional support.

By practicing self-compassion and mindfulness, you can begin to break the cycle of binge eating and regain control over your eating habits. Remember, you deserve to treat yourself with kindness and understanding, even when you make mistakes. You are not alone in this journey, and with self-compassion, you can overcome out of control eating and create a healthier relationship with food.

Chapter 6: Creating a Balanced Relationship with Food

Ditching Restrictive Diets

For those struggling with out of control eating, the idea of following a restrictive diet may seem like the perfect solution. However, the truth is that restrictive diets often do more harm than good in the long run. These diets can lead to feelings of deprivation, which can ultimately trigger binge eating episodes.

In order to break free from the cycle of binge eating, it is important to ditch restrictive diets and instead focus on building a healthy relationship with food. This means listening to your body's hunger and fullness cues, rather than following strict rules about what you can and cannot eat.

One way to do this is to practice mindful eating. This involves paying attention to the taste, texture, and sensations of each bite of food, rather than mindlessly consuming large quantities without really tasting or enjoying them. By slowing down and savoring your food, you can begin to tune into your body's signals of hunger and fullness, helping you to eat in a more balanced and satisfying way.

It is also important to remember that food is not the enemy. It is essential for nourishing our bodies and providing us with the energy we need to live our lives to the fullest. By shifting your mindset from viewing food as the enemy to seeing it as a source of nourishment and pleasure, you can begin to break free from the cycle of binge eating.

In conclusion, ditching restrictive diets is a crucial step in overcoming out of control eating. By focusing on building a healthy relationship with food and practicing mindful eating, you can begin to regain control over your eating habits and break free from the cycle of binge eating. Remember, you are not alone in this journey, and there is help available to support you every step of the way.

Finding Joy in Nourishing Your Body

Finding joy in nourishing your body is a crucial step in overcoming out of control eating habits. For many people who struggle with binge eating in solitude, the act of mindlessly consuming food can feel like a source of comfort or escape. However, it is important to recognize that true joy and fulfillment come from taking care of our bodies in a healthy and sustainable way.

One way to begin finding joy in nourishing your body is to shift your perspective on food. Instead of viewing food as a source of guilt or shame, try to see it as fuel for your body and a means of self-care. By choosing nutritious and satisfying foods, you can nourish your body and mind, leading to increased energy, improved mood, and better overall health.

Another important aspect of finding joy in nourishing your body is to practice mindfulness while eating. This means being fully present and aware of what you are consuming, savoring each bite and paying attention to how different foods make you feel. By tuning into your body's hunger and fullness cues, you can begin to eat more intuitively and break free from the cycle of mindless eating.

In addition to mindful eating, incorporating regular physical activity into your routine can also help you connect with your body and foster a sense of well-being. Exercise not only boosts your mood and energy levels but also helps you build a positive relationship with your body, making you more mindful of the choices you make when it comes to nourishment.

By finding joy in nourishing your body, you can begin to break free from the cycle of out of control eating and create a healthier, more balanced relationship with food. Remember, you deserve to treat your body with kindness and respect, and by prioritizing self-care and nourishment, you can take the first steps towards overcoming binge eating and reclaiming control over your eating habits.

Cultivating a Positive Body Image

Cultivating a positive body image is crucial for individuals who struggle with binge eating and feel out of control when it comes to their eating habits. It is common for those who experience this to have negative feelings towards their bodies, which can contribute to the cycle of binge eating. By focusing on developing a positive body image, individuals can begin to break free from the harmful patterns of overeating and learn to nourish their bodies in a more mindful way.

One way to cultivate a positive body image is to practice self-compassion. It is important for individuals to be kind to themselves and treat themselves with the same love and respect that they would show to a friend. This can involve reframing negative thoughts about one's body and focusing on the positive aspects of themselves.

Another important aspect of developing a positive body image is to engage in activities that make you feel good about yourself. This could include exercise, spending time with loved ones, or pursuing hobbies that bring joy and fulfillment. By focusing on activities that make you feel good, you can begin to shift your mindset away from negative body image thoughts.

Additionally, seeking support from a therapist or support group can be incredibly beneficial for individuals struggling with binge eating. Talking to a professional or others who have experienced similar struggles can provide valuable insight and guidance on how to overcome binge eating behaviors.

Overall, cultivating a positive body image is a key component in breaking the cycle of binge eating. By practicing self-compassion, engaging in activities that bring joy, and seeking support, individuals can begin to develop a healthier relationship with food and their bodies.

Chapter 7: Maintaining Progress and Preventing Relapse

Identifying Triggers and Warning Signs

For those struggling with out-of-control eating, it can be overwhelming to try and understand why you feel compelled to eat uncontrollably. However, recognizing your triggers and warning signs is a crucial step in breaking the cycle of binge eating and regaining control over your relationship with food.

Triggers can vary from person to person, but common ones include stress, boredom, loneliness, and even certain emotions such as sadness or anger. By identifying what triggers your urge to overeat, you can start to develop coping strategies to address those underlying issues instead of turning to food for comfort.

Warning signs are often physical or emotional cues that indicate you are about to engage in a binge eating episode. These can include feeling out of control around food, eating rapidly or in secret, and experiencing guilt or shame after eating. By becoming more aware of these warning signs, you can intervene before a binge occurs and take steps to prevent it.

One helpful strategy for identifying triggers and warning signs is to keep a food journal. Write down what you eat, when you eat, how you feel before and after eating, and any thoughts or emotions that may have contributed to your eating behavior. This can help you identify patterns and gain insight into the root causes of your binge eating.

Additionally, seeking support from a therapist, counselor, or support group can be instrumental in helping you identify and address your triggers and warning signs. Having someone to talk to about your struggles can provide valuable perspective and guidance as you work towards breaking free from out-of-control eating.

Remember, you are not alone in your battle with binge eating. By taking the time to identify your triggers and warning signs, you can begin to understand your relationship with food and take steps towards healing and recovery.

Strategies for Managing Cravings

When it comes to managing cravings and breaking the binge eating cycle, there are several effective strategies that can help individuals regain control over their eating habits. For those who struggle with mindlessly consuming large quantities of food when alone and feeling out of control, it's important to recognize that help is available and that change is possible.

One key strategy for managing cravings is to identify triggers that lead to binge eating episodes. This could be stress, boredom, loneliness, or certain emotions that trigger the desire to eat uncontrollably. By identifying these triggers, individuals can develop alternative coping mechanisms to deal with these emotions in a healthier way, such as practicing mindfulness, engaging in physical activity, or seeking support from a therapist or support group.

Another important strategy is to establish a structured eating routine. This includes eating regular meals and snacks throughout the day to prevent extreme hunger, which can often lead to overeating. Planning meals ahead of time and keeping healthy snacks on hand can help reduce the temptation to binge on unhealthy foods.

Additionally, it can be helpful to practice mindful eating, which involves being fully present and aware of the eating experience. This means eating slowly, savoring each bite, and paying attention to hunger and fullness cues. By tuning into the body's signals, individuals can better regulate their food intake and avoid overeating.

Lastly, seeking professional help from a therapist, nutritionist, or support group can provide valuable guidance and support in overcoming binge eating behaviors. It's important for individuals to know that they are not alone in their struggles and that there are resources available to help them break free from the cycle of out of control eating.

By implementing these strategies and seeking support, individuals can begin to take control of their cravings and develop healthier eating habits that promote overall well-being and balance.

Celebrating Successes and Learning from Setbacks

In the journey to overcome out of control eating, it is important to celebrate successes, no matter how small, and learn from setbacks along the way. This subchapter will explore the significance of acknowledging achievements and using setbacks as opportunities for growth and progress.

Celebrating successes is crucial in the recovery process. Whether it's being able to resist a binge urge, making healthier food choices, or practicing mindful eating, each victory should be acknowledged and celebrated. By recognizing these achievements, individuals can boost their self-esteem and motivation to continue making positive changes in their eating habits.

However, setbacks are inevitable in the journey to overcoming out of control eating. It's important to view setbacks not as failures, but as learning experiences. By reflecting on what triggered the setback and identifying strategies to prevent it from happening again, individuals can gain valuable insights into their eating patterns and behaviors.

One helpful tip is to keep a journal to track both successes and setbacks. By writing down thoughts, emotions, and behaviors related to eating, individuals can better understand their triggers and develop strategies to overcome them. Additionally, seeking support from a therapist, support group, or loved ones can provide encouragement and guidance during challenging times.

Overall, celebrating successes and learning from setbacks are essential components of breaking the binge eating cycle. By acknowledging achievements and using setbacks as opportunities for growth, individuals can develop a healthier relationship with food and regain control over their eating habits. Remember, progress is not linear, and it's okay to stumble along the way. What matters most is the willingness to learn, grow, and continue moving forward towards a healthier, happier life.

Chapter 8: Supporting a Loved One with Binge Eating Disorder

Educating Yourself on Binge Eating

Understanding the root causes and triggers of binge eating is crucial in order to overcome this destructive behavior. If you find yourself constantly consuming large amounts of food in secret, feeling shame and guilt afterwards, you may be struggling with binge eating disorder. But fear not, there is hope and help available to break free from this cycle of out-of-control eating.

One of the first steps in educating yourself on binge eating is to recognize the signs and symptoms. This includes eating large quantities of food in a short period of time, feeling a loss of control during episodes of binge eating, and experiencing shame or guilt afterwards. It is important to be aware of these warning signs so that you can seek help and support from professionals who specialize in treating binge eating disorder.

Another important aspect of educating yourself on binge eating is to understand the emotional and psychological factors that contribute to this behavior. Binge eating is often a coping mechanism for dealing with difficult emotions such as stress, anxiety, loneliness, or depression. By addressing these underlying issues and finding healthier ways to cope with emotions, you can begin to break free from the cycle of binge eating.

Seeking support from a therapist, counselor, or support group can also be beneficial in educating yourself on binge eating. These professionals can provide you with the tools and strategies needed to overcome binge eating, as well as offer a safe space to explore the underlying issues that may be driving this behavior.

Remember, you are not alone in your struggle with binge eating. By educating yourself on this disorder and seeking help from professionals, you can take the first step towards breaking free from the cycle of out-of-control eating and reclaiming control over your relationship with food.

Offering Non-Judgmental Support

One of the most important aspects of helping someone who struggles with out of control eating is providing non-judgmental support. It can be incredibly difficult for individuals to open up about their struggles with food, especially if they feel ashamed or embarrassed. By offering a safe and supportive environment, you can help create a space where they feel comfortable talking about their challenges and seeking help.

When offering non-judgmental support, it's important to listen without passing judgment or offering unsolicited advice. Instead, focus on being a compassionate and empathetic listener, validating their feelings and experiences. Let them know that you are there to support them, no matter what they are going through.

Avoid making negative comments or criticizing their eating habits, as this can further exacerbate feelings of shame and guilt. Instead, focus on encouraging positive behaviors and offering reassurance that change is possible with the right support and resources.

It's also important to respect their boundaries and not push them to change before they are ready. Remember, everyone's journey to overcoming out of control eating is unique, and progress may take time. Be patient and supportive, and let them know that you are there for them whenever they are ready to make changes.

In conclusion, offering non-judgmental support is essential in helping individuals who struggle with out of control eating. By creating a safe and supportive environment, you can help them feel heard, understood, and empowered to make positive changes in their relationship with food. Together, we can break the cycle of binge eating and help individuals regain control over their eating habits.

Encouraging Professional Help if Needed

Seeking professional help is a crucial step in overcoming out of control eating habits. If you find yourself constantly eating mindlessly, feeling like you have no control over your eating, and doing so in secrecy, it may be time to reach out for support.

Many people struggling with binge eating or out of control eating feel ashamed or embarrassed to seek help. However, it is essential to remember that you are not alone in this struggle, and there are professionals who are trained to help you through it.

Therapists, counselors, and nutritionists specializing in eating disorders can provide valuable support and guidance as you work towards breaking the binge cycle. They can help you identify triggers for your overeating, develop coping strategies, and create a balanced eating plan that works for you.

Support groups and online forums can also be helpful in connecting with others who are going through similar experiences. Sharing your thoughts and feelings with others who understand can provide a sense of community and reduce feelings of isolation.

Remember, it takes strength and courage to ask for help, but doing so is a powerful step towards regaining control over your eating habits. Don't be afraid to reach out to a professional for support – you deserve to live a life free from the constant cycle of binge eating.

Chapter 9: Living a Life Free from Binge Eating

Finding Fulfillment Beyond Food

In the journey to overcome out of control eating and binge eating, it is crucial to explore ways to find fulfillment beyond food. Many people who struggle with these issues often turn to food as a source of comfort, distraction, or escape. However, relying solely on food to fulfill emotional needs can lead to a cycle of guilt, shame, and ultimately, more overeating.

One key step in breaking the binge cycle is to identify and address the underlying emotions that drive the urge to overeat. By becoming more aware of these emotions, individuals can begin to develop healthier coping strategies that do not involve food. This may involve seeking support from a therapist, joining a support group, or practicing mindfulness and stress-reducing techniques.

Additionally, finding activities and hobbies that bring joy and fulfillment can help fill the void that food may be temporarily filling. Engaging in regular physical activity, pursuing creative outlets, or volunteering for a cause can provide a sense of purpose and satisfaction that goes beyond the momentary pleasure of eating.

It is also important to cultivate a positive body image and practice self-care. Learning to appreciate and respect your body for all that it does for you can shift the focus away from food and towards nourishing and caring for yourself in a holistic way.

By finding fulfillment beyond food, individuals can begin to break free from the cycle of out of control eating and reclaim control over their relationship with food. It is a journey that requires patience, self-compassion, and a willingness to explore new ways of finding satisfaction and joy in life.

Embracing Self-Care and Self-Love

Embracing self-care and self-love is essential for those struggling with binge eating and out of control eating. It may seem counterintuitive to focus on yourself when you feel like your eating habits are spiraling out of control, but prioritizing your own well-being is key to breaking the cycle of mindless eating.

One of the first steps towards overcoming binge eating is learning to listen to your body and recognizing the difference between physical hunger and emotional hunger. By practicing mindfulness and paying attention to the signals your body is sending, you can begin to address the root causes of your out of control eating habits.

Self-care activities such as meditation, yoga, or journaling can help you develop a deeper connection with yourself and better understand your triggers for binge eating. Taking time for self-reflection and introspection can also help you build a healthier relationship with food and break free from the cycle of mindless eating.

Self-love is another crucial component of overcoming binge eating. Learning to accept and appreciate yourself unconditionally, regardless of your eating habits, is essential for building a positive self-image and fostering a sense of self-worth. By practicing self-compassion and treating yourself with kindness and understanding, you can begin to heal the emotional wounds that may be driving your out of control eating.

Incorporating self-care and self-love practices into your daily routine can provide you with the tools and support you need to break free from the cycle of binge eating. Remember, you are worthy of love and care, and by prioritizing your own well-being, you can begin to take control of your eating habits and live a more fulfilling and balanced life.

Moving Forward with Confidence and Resilience

So you've recognized that you have a problem with out-of-control eating, and you're ready to take the first steps towards overcoming it. Congratulations on taking this important first step towards regaining control of your eating habits. It's not an easy journey, but with dedication, patience, and the right strategies, you can break free from the cycle of binge eating.

One of the key factors in moving forward with confidence and resilience is to understand that you are not alone in this struggle. Many people battle with out-of-control eating, often in silence and isolation. It's important to reach out for support, whether that's through a therapist, a support group, or trusted friends and family members. Sharing your struggles with others can help lighten the burden and provide you with the encouragement and accountability you need to make positive changes.

Another important aspect of moving forward is to develop healthy coping mechanisms for dealing with stress, emotions, and other triggers that may lead to binge eating episodes. This could include practicing mindfulness, engaging in regular physical activity, journaling, or finding creative outlets for expressing your emotions.

It's also essential to work on building resilience and self-compassion. Remember that setbacks are a natural part of the recovery process, and it's important not to beat yourself up if you slip up. Instead, focus on what you can learn from the experience and use it as an opportunity to grow stronger and more resilient.

By taking small, consistent steps towards change, seeking support, developing healthy coping mechanisms, and practicing self-compassion, you can move forward with confidence and resilience on your journey towards breaking free from out-of-control eating. Remember, you are capable of overcoming this challenge, and you deserve to live a life free from the grips of binge eating.

Appendix: Additional Resources for Help and Support

In this appendix, we provide additional resources for individuals struggling with binge eating and out of control eating. If you find yourself unable to stop eating, whether it be in secret or alone, it's important to know that you are not alone in this struggle. There are resources available to help you regain control over your eating habits and develop a healthier relationship with food.

One of the first resources we recommend is seeking support from a therapist or counselor who specializes in disordered eating. Talking to a professional can help you understand the root causes of your binge eating behavior and develop coping strategies to overcome it. Additionally, joining a support group for individuals with similar struggles can provide a sense of community and understanding.

For those looking for more structured help, there are many treatment programs and clinics that specialize in treating binge eating disorder and other forms of disordered eating. These programs often include therapy, nutrition counseling, and support groups to help individuals address their eating habits and develop healthier behaviors.

In addition to professional help, there are also a number of self-help books and online resources available for individuals struggling with binge eating. These resources can provide valuable information and strategies for overcoming binge eating behaviors and developing a healthier relationship with food.

Remember, it's important to reach out for help and support if you find yourself unable to stop eating. You deserve to live a life free from the cycle of binge eating, and there are resources available to help you on your journey to recovery.